DR. BARBARA O'NEILL'S SLOW COOKER COOKBOOK

Enjoy fast and easy 365day nutrious recipes to stay healthy with 30day meal plan to renew your body systems.

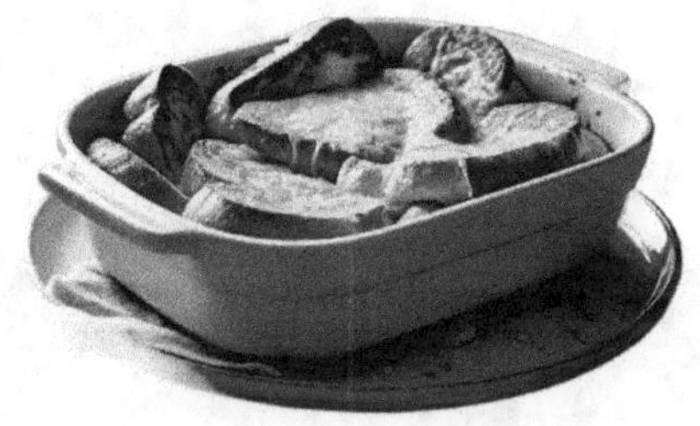

Dr. D. SAM

TABLE OF CONTENT

INTRODUCTION

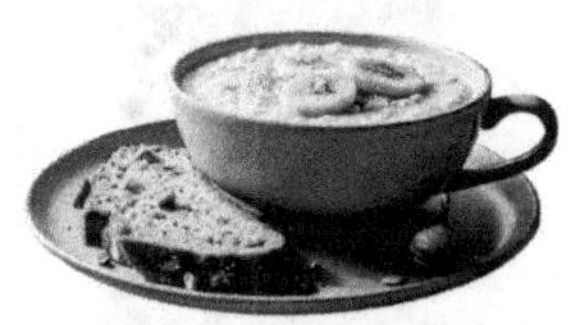

Introducing Dr. Barbara O'Neill's Slow Cooker Cookbook, a culinary companion designed to simplify mealtime without compromising on flavor or nutrition. Packed with an array of tantalizing recipes, this cookbook offers a diverse range of dishes, from savory soups and hearty stews to delectable desserts, all crafted to perfection in the convenience of your slow cooker. Dr. O'Neill's expertise in health and nutrition shines through each recipe, ensuring that every bite is not only delicious but also nourishing. Say goodbye to kitchen stress and hello to effortless, wholesome cooking with Dr. Barbara O'Neill's Slow Cooker Cookbook."

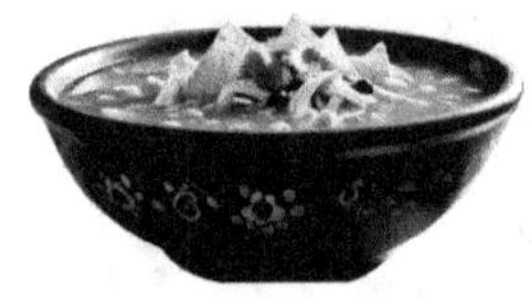

WHAT DR. BARBARA O'NEILL'S MEANS.

Dr. Barbara O'Neill is a researcher, lecturer, and specialist in nutrition, health, and personal finance. She is well-known for her contributions to financial education, especially in the fields of debt management, investing, saving, and budgeting. She frequently focuses on providing practical advice and education to enable people and families to enhance their financial well-being. O'Neill also advocates for holistic wellness and healthy lifestyle choices, drawing on his extensive knowledge in nutrition and health. She has received widespread recognition for her writing, teaching, and public speaking contributions to these subjects.

ADVANTAGES OF DR. BARBARA O'NEILL

Dr. Barbara O'Neill's knowledge in nutrition, health, and personal finance benefits people and communities in many ways.

Education: O'Neill equips people with the information and abilities necessary to make wise decisions by offering easily available and useful instruction on nutrition, health, and personal finance.

Financial Literacy: By assisting people in gaining good financial literacy skills, such as debt management, budgeting, saving, and investing, she helps them achieve more financial security and stability.

wellbeing Promotion: By highlighting the connection between one's physical and financial well-being, O'Neill encourages holistic wellbeing. Her advice inspires others to lead healthy lifestyles that improve their general well-being.

Empowerment: O'Neill develops a sense of confidence and self-reliance in her students by giving them the tools and resources they need to take charge of their health and money.

Research and Expertise: O'Neill's work as a researcher enriches the body of knowledge and informs best practices in the areas of nutrition, health, and personal finance.

Impact on Communities: Her work helps communities as a whole, fostering better health outcomes, financial stability, and a higher standard of living.

Advocacy: O'Neill works to provide conditions that promote everyone's access to good financial and health outcomes by supporting laws and programs that promote financial wellness and education.

Inspiration: O'Neill encourages others to prioritize their financial and health goals by her enthusiasm, commitment, and helpful counsel, bringing about positive change in their lives and communities.

Overall, Dr. Barbara O'Neill's work has many positive effects that touch the lives of both individuals and communities through advocacy, empowerment, and education.

MEALS TO CONSUME AT DR. BARBARA O'NEILL

A healthy, well-balanced diet is recommended by Dr. Barbara O'Neill as it promotes general health and wellness.

Although dietary demands and preferences may influence specific food choices, the following broad concepts of good eating are consistent with her teachings:

Whole Grains: Include whole grains in your diet, such as quinoa, brown rice, oats, and whole wheat bread. These aid to balance blood sugar levels and include fiber, vitamins, and minerals.

Fruits and veggies: At each meal, try to put half of your plate full with different, vibrant fruits and veggies. They enhance immune system performance and general health since they are high in vitamins, minerals, antioxidants, and fiber.

Lean Proteins: Opt for lean protein sources including beans, fish, tofu, skinless chicken, and lentils. They supply the necessary amino acids for muscle growth and repair without having too much saturated fat.

Good Fats: Include foods like avocados, almonds, seeds, and olive oil in your diet as sources of good fats. The creation of hormones, the health of the brain, and the absorption of fat-soluble vitamins all depend on these fats.

Dairy or Dairy Alternatives: Include dairy products or dairy substitutes that have been fortified with vitamin D and calcium, like yogurt, milk, or plant-based milk.

Eat Less Processed Foods and Added Sugars: Reduce your intake of foods that are high in processed components, refined grains, and added sugars. Whenever possible, choose whole, minimally processed foods.

Hydration: To stay hydrated, sip lots of water throughout the day. Limit your intake of sugar-filled beverages and caffeine.

Balance and Moderation: Make mindful of portion sizes and use restraint when selecting foods. Savor a range of dishes in sensible portion sizes to satisfy your dietary requirements without going overboard.

Keep in mind that dietary requirements could differ for each person depending on their age, gender, degree of exercise, and any particular medical issues. It's crucial to speak with a medical expert or registered dietitian for individualized, needs-based nutrition guidance.

FOOD TO EAT IN DR. BARBARA O'NEILL'S

Although I am not aware of Dr. Barbara O'Neill's exact dietary preferences, I can recommend items that are consistent with the broad health and nutrition principles that she probably supports:

Whole Foods: Make up a large portion of your diet of whole, minimally processed foods. Fruits, vegetables, whole grains, lean meats, and good fats are all included in this.

Fruits and veggies: Stimulate your meals and snacks with a range of vibrant fruits and veggies. These are high in fiber, antioxidants, minerals, and vitamins.

Whole Grains: Opt for whole grains including whole wheat bread, quinoa, brown rice, oats, and barley. They include fiber, complex carbs, and vital minerals.

Lean Proteins: Consume lean protein-rich foods including fish, beans, lentils, tofu, tempeh, and fowl (without the skin). These are crucial for the development, maintenance, and general health of muscles.

Good Fats: Include foods like avocados, nuts, seeds, olive oil, and fatty fish like trout and salmon in your diet. These are good sources of fat. These fats are good for hormone balance, heart health, and brain function.

Dairy or Dairy Alternatives: If you can handle it, go for dairy-free or low-fat items like cheese, yogurt, and milk. For people who cannot digest lactose or would rather consume plant-based foods, you may want to look into dairy-free yogurts or fortified plant milks like soy or almond milk.

Hydration: To stay hydrated, sip lots of water throughout the day. Infused water and herbal teas can also be cooling choices.

Portion Control and Balance: Make balanced, moderate eating choices. Aim for a balanced intake of carbohydrates, proteins, and fats while paying attention to portion sizes.

Individual dietary requirements and preferences can differ, so it's important to pay attention to your body's signals and make decisions that promote your general health and wellbeing. See a qualified dietitian or other healthcare provider for individualized advice if you have any particular dietary questions or medical issues.

Overnight Oats:

- Ingredients:
    1. 1 cup rolled oats
    2. 2 cups milk (dairy or plant-based)
    3. 2 tablespoons honey or maple syrup
    4. 1 teaspoon vanilla extract
    5. Optional toppings: sliced fruits, nuts, seeds
- Instructions:
    1. In the slow cooker, combine oats, milk, honey

(or maple syrup), and vanilla extract. Stir well.
2. Cover and cook on low for 6-8 hours or overnight.
3. Serve warm, topped with your favorite fruits, nuts, or seeds.

Vegetable Frittata:

- Ingredients:
    1. 8 eggs
    2. 1 cup chopped vegetables (bell peppers, onions, spinach, mushrooms, etc.)
    3. 1/2 cup shredded cheese
    4. Salt and pepper to taste
- Instructions:
    1. Grease the slow cooker insert with cooking spray or butter.
    2. In a bowl, beat the eggs and season with salt and pepper.

3. Stir in the chopped vegetables and shredded cheese.
4. Pour the egg mixture into the slow cooker.
5. Cover and cook on low for 2-3 hours or until the frittata is set.
6. Slice and serve warm.

Slow Cooker Breakfast Casserole:

- Ingredients:
    1. 6 slices bacon, cooked and crumbled
    2. 4 cups frozen hash browns
    3. 1 cup shredded cheddar cheese
    4. 6 eggs
    5. 1/2 cup milk
    6. Salt and pepper to taste
- Instructions:
    1. Layer half of the hash browns, bacon, and cheese in the greased slow cooker.

2. Repeat with another layer of hash browns, bacon, and cheese.
3. In a separate bowl, whisk together eggs, milk, salt, and pepper.
4. Pour the egg mixture over the layers in the slow cooker.
5. Cover and cook on low for 6-8 hours or on high for 3-4 hours, until eggs are set.
6. Serve hot.

Slow Cooker Breakfast Burritos:

- Ingredients:
    1. 8 large flour tortillas
    2. 8 eggs, scrambled
    3. 1 cup cooked breakfast sausage or bacon, crumbled
    4. 1 cup shredded cheddar cheese

5. Optional toppings: salsa, sour cream, avocado

- Instructions:
    1. Lay out tortillas and divide scrambled eggs, cooked sausage or bacon, and cheese evenly among them.
    2. Roll up the tortillas, folding in the sides to secure the filling.
    3. Place the rolled burritos seam-side down in the slow cooker.
    4. Cover and cook on low for 2-3 hours or until heated through.
    5. Serve with your favorite toppings.

Slow Cooker French Toast Casserole:

- Ingredients:
    1. 1 loaf French bread, cubed
    2. 6 eggs

3. 1 1/2 cups milk
4. 1/4 cup maple syrup
5. 1 teaspoon vanilla extract
6. 1 teaspoon ground cinnamon
7. 1/2 teaspoon ground nutmeg

- Instructions:
    1. Grease the slow cooker insert with butter.
    2. Place the cubed French bread in the slow cooker.
    3. In a bowl, whisk together eggs, milk, maple syrup, vanilla extract, cinnamon, and nutmeg.
    4. Pour the egg mixture over the bread cubes, ensuring all bread is soaked.
    5. Cover and cook on low for 3-4 hours or until set.
    6. Serve warm, optionally topped with additional

maple syrup or powdered
sugar.

Slow Cooker Breakfast Quinoa:

- Ingredients:
    1. 1 cup quinoa, rinsed
    2. 2 cups milk (dairy or plant-based)
    3. 1/4 cup honey or maple syrup
    4. 1 teaspoon vanilla extract
    5. 1/2 teaspoon ground cinnamon
    6. 1/4 cup dried fruit (such as raisins or cranberries)
    7. 1/4 cup chopped nuts (such as almonds or walnuts)
- Instructions:
    1. In the slow cooker, combine quinoa, milk, honey (or maple syrup), vanilla extract, and cinnamon. Stir well.

2. Add dried fruit and nuts, stirring to distribute evenly.
3. Cover and cook on low for 4-6 hours or on high for 2-3 hours, until quinoa is tender and most of the liquid is absorbed.
4. Serve warm, optionally topped with additional nuts or a drizzle of honey.

Slow Cooker Breakfast Cobbler:

- Ingredients:
    1. 4 cups mixed berries (such as strawberries, blueberries, and raspberries)
    2. 1/4 cup granulated sugar
    3. 1 tablespoon lemon juice
    4. 1 cup rolled oats
    5. 1/2 cup flour
    6. 1/4 cup brown sugar
    7. 1/4 cup cold butter, cubed

- Instructions:
    1. In the slow cooker, toss mixed berries with granulated sugar and lemon juice.
    2. In a separate bowl, combine oats, flour, and brown sugar. Cut in the cold butter until the mixture resembles coarse crumbs.
    3. Sprinkle the oat mixture over the berries in the slow cooker.
    4. Cover and cook on low for 3-4 hours or until the fruit is bubbling and the topping is golden brown.
    5. Serve warm, optionally topped with vanilla ice cream or whipped cream.

Slow Cooker Breakfast Tacos:

- Ingredients:

1. 8 small flour tortillas
2. 8 eggs, scrambled
3. 1 cup cooked black beans
4. 1 cup salsa
5. 1 avocado, sliced
6. 1/2 cup shredded cheese
7. Fresh cilantro, chopped (for garnish)

- Instructions:
  1. Warm tortillas in the microwave or on a skillet.
  2. Fill each tortilla with scrambled eggs, black beans, salsa, avocado slices, and shredded cheese.
  3. Roll up the tortillas to form tacos.
  4. Place the tacos in the slow cooker, seam-side down.
  5. Cover and cook on low for 1-2 hours or until heated through.

6. Serve hot, garnished with chopped cilantro.

Slow Cooker Banana Bread Oatmeal:

- Ingredients:
    1. 2 cups steel-cut oats
    2. 4 cups water
    3. 2 cups milk (dairy or plant-based)
    4. 2 ripe bananas, mashed
    5. 1/4 cup maple syrup
    6. 1 teaspoon vanilla extract
    7. 1 teaspoon ground cinnamon
    8. Pinch of salt
- Instructions:
    1. In the slow cooker, combine steel-cut oats, water, milk, mashed bananas, maple syrup, vanilla extract, cinnamon, and salt. Stir well.
    2. Cover and cook on low for 6-8 hours or overnight.

3. Stir the oatmeal before serving. If desired, top with additional sliced bananas, a drizzle of maple syrup, or a sprinkle of cinnamon.

Slow Cooker Breakfast Hash:

- Ingredients:
    1. 1 pound potatoes, diced
    2. 1 onion, chopped
    3. 1 bell pepper, diced
    4. 1 cup cooked breakfast sausage, diced
    5. 1 cup shredded cheddar cheese
    6. 6 eggs
    7. Salt and pepper to taste
- Instructions:
    1. Grease the slow cooker insert with cooking spray or butter.
    2. Layer potatoes, onion, bell pepper, cooked sausage,

and shredded cheese in the slow cooker.

3. In a bowl, beat the eggs and season with salt and pepper.
4. Pour the beaten eggs over the layers in the slow cooker.
5. Cover and cook on low for 6-8 hours or on high for 3-4 hours, until eggs are set and potatoes are tender.
6. Serve hot, optionally topped with salsa or hot sauce.

LUNCH RECIPES

Slow Cooker Chicken Tortilla Soup:

- Ingredients:
  1. 1 pound boneless, skinless chicken breasts
  2. 1 onion, diced

3. 2 cloves garlic, minced
4. 1 bell pepper, diced
5. 1 can (14.5 oz) diced tomatoes
6. 1 can (15 oz) black beans, drained and rinsed
7. 1 can (15 oz) corn kernels, drained
8. 4 cups chicken broth
9. 1 teaspoon ground cumin
10. 1 teaspoon chili powder
11. Salt and pepper to taste
12. Tortilla strips, avocado, shredded cheese, and lime wedges for serving (optional)

- Instructions:
  1. Place chicken breasts in the bottom of the slow cooker.
  2. Add diced onion, minced garlic, diced bell pepper, diced tomatoes, black beans, corn kernels,

chicken broth, ground cumin, chili powder, salt, and pepper to the slow cooker.

3. Stir to combine ingredients.
4. Cover and cook on low for 6-8 hours or on high for 3-4 hours, until chicken is cooked through and flavors are well blended.
5. Shred the chicken using two forks.
6. Serve hot, garnished with tortilla strips, avocado slices, shredded cheese, and lime wedges if desired.

Slow Cooker Beef Stew:

- Ingredients:
  1. 1.5 pounds beef stew meat, cubed
  2. 4 carrots, peeled and sliced

3. 3 potatoes, peeled and cubed
4. 1 onion, diced
5. 2 cloves garlic, minced
6. 4 cups beef broth
7. 2 tablespoons tomato paste
8. 1 teaspoon dried thyme
9. 1 teaspoon dried rosemary
10. Salt and pepper to taste
11. 2 tablespoons cornstarch (optional, for thickening)

- Instructions:
    1. Place beef stew meat, carrots, potatoes, diced onion, minced garlic, beef broth, tomato paste, dried thyme, dried rosemary, salt, and pepper in the slow cooker.
    2. Stir to combine ingredients.
    3. Cover and cook on low for 8-10 hours or on high for

4-6 hours, until beef and vegetables are tender.

4. If desired, mix cornstarch with a small amount of water to create a slurry. Stir the slurry into the stew to thicken the broth.

5. Serve hot, optionally garnished with chopped fresh parsley.

Slow Cooker Vegetarian Chili:

- Ingredients:
  1. 2 cans (15 oz each) kidney beans, drained and rinsed
  2. 1 can (15 oz) black beans, drained and rinsed
  3. 1 can (14.5 oz) diced tomatoes
  4. 1 onion, diced
  5. 1 bell pepper, diced
  6. 2 cloves garlic, minced
  7. 2 cups vegetable broth
  8. 1 tablespoon chili powder

9. 1 teaspoon ground cumin
10. 1 teaspoon smoked paprika
11. Salt and pepper to taste
- Instructions:
  1. Place kidney beans, black beans, diced tomatoes, diced onion, diced bell pepper, minced garlic, vegetable broth, chili powder, ground cumin, smoked paprika, salt, and pepper in the slow cooker.
  2. Stir to combine ingredients.
  3. Cover and cook on low for 6-8 hours or on high for 3-4 hours, until flavors are well blended.
  4. Serve hot, optionally garnished with shredded cheese, sour cream, or sliced green onions.

Slow Cooker Lentil Soup:

- Ingredients:
    1. 2 cups dry green or brown lentils, rinsed and drained
    2. 1 onion, diced
    3. 2 carrots, peeled and sliced
    4. 2 celery stalks, sliced
    5. 2 cloves garlic, minced
    6. 6 cups vegetable broth
    7. 1 can (14.5 oz) diced tomatoes
    8. 1 teaspoon dried thyme
    9. 1 teaspoon ground cumin
    10. Salt and pepper to taste
    11. Fresh lemon juice (optional, for serving)
- Instructions:
    1. Place lentils, diced onion, sliced carrots, sliced celery, minced garlic, vegetable broth, diced tomatoes, dried thyme, ground cumin, salt, and pepper in the slow cooker.

2. Stir to combine ingredients.
3. Cover and cook on low for 6-8 hours or on high for 3-4 hours, until lentils are tender.
4. Serve hot, optionally with a squeeze of fresh lemon juice.

Slow Cooker BBQ Pulled Pork Sandwiches:

- Ingredients:
    1. 3 pounds pork shoulder or butt roast
    2. 1 onion, sliced
    3. 1 cup BBQ sauce
    4. 1/2 cup apple cider vinegar
    5. 1/4 cup brown sugar
    6. 1 tablespoon Worcestershire sauce
    7. 1 teaspoon garlic powder
    8. 1 teaspoon smoked paprika

9. Salt and pepper to taste
10. Hamburger buns, coleslaw, and pickles for serving

- Instructions:
    1. Place sliced onion in the bottom of the slow cooker.
    2. Season pork roast with salt, pepper, garlic powder, and smoked paprika. Place the seasoned pork roast on top of the onions in the slow cooker.
    3. In a bowl, mix together BBQ sauce, apple cider vinegar, brown sugar, and Worcestershire sauce. Pour the mixture over the pork roast.
    4. Cover and cook on low for 8-10 hours or on high for 4-6 hours, until the pork is tender and easily shreds with a fork.

5. Shred the pork using two forks and mix it with the sauce in the slow cooker.

6. Serve the pulled pork on hamburger buns, topped with coleslaw and pickles if desired.

Slow Cooker Chicken and Rice Casserole:

- Ingredients:
  1. 1.5 pounds boneless, skinless chicken breasts, diced
  2. 1 cup long-grain white rice
  3. 1 onion, diced
  4. 2 cloves garlic, minced
  5. 1 bell pepper, diced
  6. 1 cup chicken broth
  7. 1 cup diced tomatoes
  8. 1 teaspoon dried oregano
  9. 1 teaspoon dried basil
  10. Salt and pepper to taste

11. 1 cup shredded mozzarella cheese

- Instructions:
    1. In the slow cooker, combine diced chicken breasts, white rice, diced onion, minced garlic, diced bell pepper, chicken broth, diced tomatoes, dried oregano, dried basil, salt, and pepper.
    2. Stir to combine ingredients.
    3. Cover and cook on low for 6-8 hours or on high for 3-4 hours, until the chicken is cooked through and the rice is tender.
    4. Sprinkle shredded mozzarella cheese over the chicken and rice mixture.
    5. Cover and cook for an additional 10-15 minutes, until the cheese is melted.

6. Serve hot.

Slow Cooker Minestrone Soup:

- Ingredients:
    1. 2 carrots, peeled and sliced
    2. 2 celery stalks, sliced
    3. 1 onion, diced
    4. 2 cloves garlic, minced
    5. 1 can (14.5 oz) diced tomatoes
    6. 1 can (15 oz) kidney beans, drained and rinsed
    7. 4 cups vegetable broth
    8. 1 teaspoon dried thyme
    9. 1 teaspoon dried oregano
    10. 1/2 cup small pasta (such as ditalini or macaroni)
    11. Salt and pepper to taste
    12. Fresh parsley, chopped (for garnish)
- Instructions:
    1. Place sliced carrots, sliced celery, diced onion,

minced garlic, diced tomatoes, kidney beans, vegetable broth, dried thyme, and dried oregano in the slow cooker.
2. Stir to combine ingredients.
3. Cover and cook on low for 6-8 hours or on high for 3-4 hours, until vegetables are tender.
4. Stir in the small pasta and continue cooking for an additional 20-30 minutes, until pasta is cooked al dente.
5. Season with salt and pepper to taste.
6. Serve hot, garnished with chopped fresh parsley.

Slow Cooker Beef and Broccoli:

○ Ingredients:

1. 1.5 pounds beef chuck roast, sliced thinly
2. 1/2 cup low-sodium soy sauce
3. 1/4 cup brown sugar
4. 2 cloves garlic, minced
5. 1 teaspoon sesame oil
6. 1 cup beef broth
7. 4 cups broccoli florets
8. 2 tablespoons cornstarch
9. Cooked white rice, for serving

- Instructions:
    1. In the slow cooker, combine thinly sliced beef chuck roast, low-sodium soy sauce, brown sugar, minced garlic, sesame oil, and beef broth.
    2. Stir to combine ingredients.
    3. Cover and cook on low for 6-8 hours or on high for

3-4 hours, until beef is tender.

4. In a small bowl, mix cornstarch with a small amount of water to create a slurry. Stir the slurry into the slow cooker to thicken the sauce.

5. Add broccoli florets to the slow cooker and cook for an additional 30 minutes, until broccoli is tender-crisp.

6. Serve hot over cooked white rice.

Slow Cooker Turkey Chili:

- Ingredients:
  1. 1 pound ground turkey
  2. 1 onion, diced
  3. 2 cloves garlic, minced
  4. 1 bell pepper, diced
  5. 1 can (14.5 oz) diced tomatoes

6. 1 can (15 oz) kidney beans, drained and rinsed
7. 1 can (15 oz) black beans, drained and rinsed
8. 2 cups chicken broth
9. 2 tablespoons chili powder
10. 1 teaspoon ground cumin
11. 1 teaspoon smoked paprika
12. Salt and pepper to taste
13. Shredded cheddar cheese and chopped green onions for serving (optional)

- Instructions:
    1. In a skillet, cook ground turkey over medium heat until browned. Drain excess fat.
    2. Transfer cooked turkey to the slow cooker.
    3. Add diced onion, minced garlic, diced bell pepper, diced tomatoes, kidney

beans, black beans, chicken broth, chili powder, ground cumin, smoked paprika, salt, and pepper to the slow cooker.

4. Stir to combine ingredients.
5. Cover and cook on low for 6-8 hours or on high for 3-4 hours, until flavors are well blended.
6. Serve hot, optionally garnished with shredded cheddar cheese and chopped green onions.

Slow Cooker Ratatouille:

- Ingredients:
  1. 1 eggplant, diced
  2. 2 zucchini, diced
  3. 1 onion, diced
  4. 2 bell peppers, diced
  5. 2 cloves garlic, minced

6. 1 can (14.5 oz) diced tomatoes
7. 2 tablespoons tomato paste
8. 1 teaspoon dried thyme
9. 1 teaspoon dried oregano
10. Salt and pepper to taste
11. Fresh basil, chopped (for garnish)

- Instructions:
    1. In the slow cooker, combine diced eggplant, diced zucchini, diced onion, diced bell peppers, minced garlic, diced tomatoes, tomato paste, dried thyme, dried oregano, salt, and pepper.
    2. Stir to combine ingredients.
    3. Cover and cook on low for 6-8 hours or on high for 3-4 hours, until vegetables are tender.

4. Serve hot, garnished with chopped fresh basil. Optionally, serve over cooked pasta or crusty bread.

DINNER RECIPES

Slow Cooker Balsamic Chicken:

- Ingredients:
    1. 4 boneless, skinless chicken breasts
    2. 1 onion, sliced
    3. 2 cloves garlic, minced
    4. 1/2 cup balsamic vinegar
    5. 1/4 cup honey
    6. 2 tablespoons olive oil
    7. 1 teaspoon dried thyme
    8. Salt and pepper to taste
    9. Fresh parsley, chopped (for garnish)
- Instructions:
    1. Place sliced onion in the bottom of the slow cooker.

2. Season chicken breasts with salt, pepper, and dried thyme. Place the seasoned chicken breasts on top of the onions in the slow cooker.
3. In a bowl, whisk together minced garlic, balsamic vinegar, honey, and olive oil. Pour the mixture over the chicken.
4. Cover and cook on low for 6-8 hours or on high for 3-4 hours, until chicken is cooked through and tender.
5. Serve hot, garnished with chopped fresh parsley.

Slow Cooker Beef Stroganoff:

- Ingredients:
  1. 1.5 pounds beef stew meat, cubed
  2. 1 onion, diced

3. 2 cloves garlic, minced
4. 8 oz mushrooms, sliced
5. 2 cups beef broth
6. 1 cup sour cream
7. 2 tablespoons all-purpose flour
8. 2 tablespoons Worcestershire sauce
9. Salt and pepper to taste
10. Cooked egg noodles or rice, for serving
11. Fresh parsley, chopped (for garnish)

- Instructions:
    1. Place beef stew meat, diced onion, minced garlic, sliced mushrooms, and beef broth in the slow cooker.
    2. Stir to combine ingredients.
    3. Cover and cook on low for 8-10 hours or on high for

4-6 hours, until beef is tender.

4. In a small bowl, mix sour cream, flour, and Worcestershire sauce until smooth. Stir the sour cream mixture into the slow cooker.

5. Cover and cook for an additional 30 minutes, until the sauce is thickened.

6. Serve hot over cooked egg noodles or rice, garnished with chopped fresh parsley.

Slow Cooker Vegetable Lasagna:

- Ingredients:
    1. 9 lasagna noodles, uncooked
    2. 2 cups marinara sauce
    3. 2 cups ricotta cheese

4. 2 cups shredded mozzarella cheese
5. 2 cups sliced vegetables (such as zucchini, bell peppers, and mushrooms)
6. 1/4 cup grated Parmesan cheese
7. Fresh basil, chopped (for garnish)

- Instructions:
    1. Spread a thin layer of marinara sauce on the bottom of the slow cooker insert.
    2. Break 3 lasagna noodles into pieces and arrange them over the sauce.
    3. Spread half of the ricotta cheese over the noodles, followed by half of the sliced vegetables and half of the shredded mozzarella cheese.

4. Repeat layering with marinara sauce, lasagna noodles, ricotta cheese, vegetables, and mozzarella cheese.
5. Top with a final layer of marinara sauce and sprinkle grated Parmesan cheese over the top.
6. Cover and cook on low for 4-6 hours or until noodles are tender.
7. Sprinkle chopped fresh basil over the lasagna before serving.

Slow Cooker Pork Carnitas:

- Ingredients:
  1. 3 pounds pork shoulder or butt roast
  2. 1 onion, sliced
  3. 4 cloves garlic, minced
  4. 1 tablespoon chili powder
  5. 1 teaspoon ground cumin

6. 1 teaspoon dried oregano
7. 1 teaspoon smoked paprika
8. Juice of 2 limes
9. Salt and pepper to taste
10. Corn tortillas, for serving
11. Sliced avocado, chopped cilantro, diced onion, lime wedges, for serving

- Instructions:
    1. Place sliced onion and minced garlic in the bottom of the slow cooker.
    2. Season pork roast with chili powder, ground cumin, dried oregano, smoked paprika, salt, and pepper. Place the seasoned pork roast on top of the onions and garlic in the slow cooker.
    3. Squeeze lime juice over the pork roast.

4. Cover and cook on low for 8-10 hours or on high for 4-6 hours, until pork is tender and easily shreds with a fork.
5. Shred the pork using two forks and mix it with the juices in the slow cooker.
6. Serve the pork carnitas in corn tortillas, topped with sliced avocado, chopped cilantro, diced onion, and lime wedges.

Slow Cooker Moroccan Chickpea Tagine:

- Ingredients:
  1. 2 cans (15 oz each) chickpeas, drained and rinsed
  2. 1 onion, diced
  3. 2 carrots, peeled and sliced
  4. 1 bell pepper, diced
  5. 2 cloves garlic, minced

6. 1 can (14.5 oz) diced tomatoes
7. 1 cup vegetable broth
8. 1 teaspoon ground cumin
9. 1 teaspoon ground coriander
10. 1 teaspoon ground cinnamon
11. 1/2 teaspoon ground ginger
12. 1/4 teaspoon cayenne pepper (optional)
13. Salt and pepper to taste
14. Cooked couscous or rice, for serving
15. Fresh cilantro, chopped (for garnish)

- Instructions:
    1. In the slow cooker, combine chickpeas, diced onion, sliced carrots, diced bell pepper, minced garlic, diced tomatoes, vegetable broth, ground cumin,

ground coriander, ground cinnamon, ground ginger, cayenne pepper (if using), salt, and pepper.
2. Stir to combine ingredients.
3. Cover and cook on low for 6-8 hours or on high for 3-4 hours, until vegetables are tender.
4. Serve hot over cooked couscous or rice, garnished with chopped fresh cilantro.

Slow Cooker Lemon Garlic Chicken:

- Ingredients:
    1. 4 boneless, skinless chicken breasts
    2. 1 lemon, juiced and zested
    3. 4 cloves garlic, minced
    4. 1/4 cup olive oil
    5. 1 teaspoon dried oregano
    6. 1/2 teaspoon dried thyme

7. Salt and pepper to taste
8. Fresh parsley, chopped (for garnish)

- Instructions:
    1. In a small bowl, whisk together lemon juice, lemon zest, minced garlic, olive oil, dried oregano, dried thyme, salt, and pepper.
    2. Place chicken breasts in the slow cooker.
    3. Pour the lemon garlic mixture over the chicken, ensuring it is well coated.
    4. Cover and cook on low for 6-8 hours or on high for 3-4 hours, until chicken is cooked through and tender.
    5. Serve hot, garnished with chopped fresh parsley.

Slow Cooker Teriyaki Beef:

- Ingredients:
    1. 2 pounds beef chuck roast, sliced thinly
    2. 1/2 cup soy sauce
    3. 1/4 cup honey
    4. 2 cloves garlic, minced
    5. 1 tablespoon grated ginger
    6. 2 tablespoons rice vinegar
    7. 1 tablespoon cornstarch
    8. 2 tablespoons water
    9. Sesame seeds and sliced green onions (for garnish)
- Instructions:
    1. In the slow cooker, combine thinly sliced beef chuck roast, soy sauce, honey, minced garlic, grated ginger, and rice vinegar.
    2. Stir to combine ingredients.
    3. Cover and cook on low for 6-8 hours or on high for

3-4 hours, until beef is tender.

4. In a small bowl, mix cornstarch with water to create a slurry. Stir the slurry into the slow cooker to thicken the sauce.

5. Serve hot, garnished with sesame seeds and sliced green onions. Optionally, serve over rice or noodles.

Slow Cooker Mediterranean Lentil Stew:

- Ingredients:
    1. 2 cups dry green or brown lentils, rinsed and drained
    2. 1 onion, diced
    3. 2 carrots, peeled and sliced
    4. 2 celery stalks, sliced
    5. 2 cloves garlic, minced
    6. 1 can (14.5 oz) diced tomatoes
    7. 4 cups vegetable broth
    8. 1 teaspoon dried oregano

9. 1 teaspoon dried basil

10. 1/2 teaspoon smoked paprika

11. Salt and pepper to taste

12. Crumbled feta cheese and chopped fresh parsley (for garnish)

- Instructions:

1. In the slow cooker, combine lentils, diced onion, sliced carrots, sliced celery, minced garlic, diced tomatoes, vegetable broth, dried oregano, dried basil, smoked paprika, salt, and pepper.

2. Stir to combine ingredients.

3. Cover and cook on low for 6-8 hours or on high for 3-4 hours, until lentils are tender.

4. Serve hot, garnished with crumbled feta cheese and chopped fresh parsley.

Slow Cooker Coconut Curry Chicken:

- Ingredients:
    1. 1.5 pounds boneless, skinless chicken thighs, cut into chunks
    2. 1 onion, diced
    3. 2 bell peppers, diced
    4. 1 cup diced potatoes
    5. 1 can (13.5 oz) coconut milk
    6. 1/4 cup red curry paste
    7. 2 tablespoons soy sauce
    8. 2 tablespoons brown sugar
    9. 2 cloves garlic, minced
    10. 1 tablespoon grated ginger
    11. 1 tablespoon lime juice
    12. Salt and pepper to taste
    13. Cooked rice, for serving

14. Chopped cilantro and lime wedges (for garnish)

- Instructions:
    1. In the slow cooker, combine chicken thighs, diced onion, diced bell peppers, diced potatoes, coconut milk, red curry paste, soy sauce, brown sugar, minced garlic, grated ginger, lime juice, salt, and pepper.
    2. Stir to combine ingredients.
    3. Cover and cook on low for 6-8 hours or on high for 3-4 hours, until chicken is cooked through and vegetables are tender.
    4. Serve hot over cooked rice, garnished with chopped cilantro and lime wedges.

Slow Cooker Mushroom Risotto:

- Ingredients:
    1. 2 cups Arborio rice
    2. 6 cups vegetable broth
    3. 1 onion, diced
    4. 2 cloves garlic, minced
    5. 8 oz mushrooms, sliced
    6. 1/2 cup dry white wine (optional)
    7. 1/2 cup grated Parmesan cheese
    8. 2 tablespoons unsalted butter
    9. Salt and pepper to taste
    10. Chopped fresh parsley (for garnish)
- Instructions:
    1. In the slow cooker, combine Arborio rice, vegetable broth, diced onion, minced garlic, and sliced mushrooms.
    2. Stir to combine ingredients.

3. Cover and cook on low for 2-3 hours, until rice is tender and creamy.
4. Stir in dry white wine (if using), grated Parmesan cheese, and unsalted butter until well combined.
5. Season with salt and pepper to taste.
6. Serve hot, garnished with chopped fresh parsley.

SNACKS RECIPES

Slow Cooker Cinnamon Almonds
Ingredients:

- 2 cups raw almonds
- 1/4 cup honey
- 1 tablespoon cinnamon
- 1/4 teaspoon salt

Instructions:

1. In a bowl, mix together honey, cinnamon, and salt.
2. Add almonds to the slow cooker and pour the honey mixture over them, stirring to coat evenly.
3. Cook on low for 2 hours, stirring occasionally.
4. Spread the almonds on a baking sheet to cool before serving.

Slow Cooker Buffalo Chicken Dip
Ingredients:

- 2 cups shredded cooked chicken
- 8 oz cream cheese, softened
- 1/2 cup buffalo sauce
- 1/2 cup ranch dressing
- 1 cup shredded cheddar cheese

Instructions:

1. In the slow cooker, combine shredded chicken, cream cheese, buffalo sauce, ranch dressing, and shredded cheddar cheese.

2. Cook on low for 1-2 hours, stirring occasionally, until the dip is heated through and the cheese is melted.
3. Serve with tortilla chips, crackers, or celery sticks.

Slow Cooker Chocolate Fondue

Ingredients:

- 12 oz chocolate chips
- 1/2 cup heavy cream
- 1 teaspoon vanilla extract
- Assorted fruits and marshmallows for dipping

Instructions:

1. In the slow cooker, combine chocolate chips, heavy cream, and vanilla extract.
2. Cook on low for 1-2 hours, stirring occasionally, until the chocolate is melted and smooth.
3. Once melted, reduce heat to warm and serve with assorted fruits and marshmallows for dipping.

Slow Cooker Spicy Nuts

Ingredients:

- 2 cups mixed nuts (such as almonds, cashews, and pecans)
- 2 tablespoons olive oil
- 1 tablespoon honey
- 1 teaspoon smoked paprika
- 1/2 teaspoon cayenne pepper
- 1/2 teaspoon garlic powder
- 1/2 teaspoon salt

Instructions:

1. In a bowl, mix together olive oil, honey, smoked paprika, cayenne pepper, garlic powder, and salt.
2. Add mixed nuts to the slow cooker and pour the spice mixture over them, stirring to coat evenly.
3. Cook on low for 2 hours, stirring occasionally.
4. Spread the nuts on a baking sheet to cool before serving.

Slow Cooker Spinach and Artichoke Dip

Ingredients:

- 8 oz cream cheese, softened
- 1/2 cup sour cream
- 1/4 cup mayonnaise
- 1/2 cup grated Parmesan cheese
- 1 cup shredded mozzarella cheese
- 1 can (14 oz) artichoke hearts, drained and chopped
- 1 cup chopped spinach (fresh or frozen)
- 2 cloves garlic, minced
- Salt and pepper to taste

Instructions:

1. In the slow cooker, combine cream cheese, sour cream, mayonnaise, Parmesan cheese, mozzarella cheese, artichoke hearts, spinach, and minced garlic.

2. Cook on low for 2 hours, stirring occasionally, until the dip is heated through and the cheeses are melted.
3. Season with salt and pepper to taste.
4. Serve with tortilla chips, crackers, or sliced baguette.

Slow Cooker BBQ Meatballs

Ingredients:

- 1 pound ground beef or turkey
- 1/2 cup breadcrumbs
- 1/4 cup milk
- 1 egg
- 1/2 cup BBQ sauce
- 1/4 cup ketchup
- 1 tablespoon Worcestershire sauce
- 1 teaspoon garlic powder
- Salt and pepper to taste

Instructions:

1. In a bowl, mix together ground beef or turkey, breadcrumbs, milk, egg, garlic powder, salt, and pepper until well

combined. Roll mixture into small meatballs.

2. In the slow cooker, combine BBQ sauce, ketchup, and Worcestershire sauce. Add meatballs to the sauce mixture, stirring to coat evenly.

3. Cook on low for 2-3 hours, stirring occasionally, until the meatballs are cooked through and the sauce is bubbly.

4. Serve with toothpicks for easy snacking.

Slow Cooker Chex Mix

Ingredients:

- 3 cups rice Chex cereal
- 3 cups corn Chex cereal
- 2 cups pretzel sticks
- 1 cup mixed nuts
- 6 tablespoons unsalted butter, melted
- 2 tablespoons Worcestershire sauce
- 1 1/2 teaspoons seasoned salt
- 3/4 teaspoon garlic powder

- 1/2 teaspoon onion powder

Instructions:

1. In the slow cooker, combine rice Chex cereal, corn Chex cereal, pretzel sticks, and mixed nuts.
2. In a small bowl, whisk together melted butter, Worcestershire sauce, seasoned salt, garlic powder, and onion powder. Pour over the cereal mixture, stirring to coat evenly.
3. Cook on low for 2-3 hours, stirring every 30 minutes, until the Chex mix is toasted and fragrant.
4. Spread the Chex mix on a baking sheet to cool before serving.

Slow Cooker S'mores Dip

Ingredients:

- 1 cup chocolate chips
- 1 cup mini marshmallows
- 1/4 cup heavy cream
- Graham crackers for dipping

Instructions:

1. In the slow cooker, combine chocolate chips, mini marshmallows, and heavy cream.
2. Cook on low for 1-2 hours, stirring occasionally, until the chocolate is melted and the mixture is smooth.
3. Once melted, reduce heat to warm and serve with graham crackers for dipping.

Slow Cooker Sweet and Spicy Chicken Wings

Ingredients:

- 2 pounds chicken wings
- 1/2 cup honey
- 1/4 cup soy sauce
- 2 tablespoons sriracha sauce
- 2 cloves garlic, minced
- 1 teaspoon grated ginger
- Sesame seeds and chopped green onions for garnish

Instructions:

1. In the slow cooker, combine honey, soy sauce, sriracha sauce, minced garlic, and grated ginger.
2. Add chicken wings to the sauce mixture, stirring to coat evenly.
3. Cook on low for 3-4 hours, or until the chicken is cooked through and tender.
4. Sprinkle with sesame seeds and chopped green onions before serving.

Slow Cooker Queso Dip

Ingredients:

- 1 pound Velveeta cheese, cubed
- 1 can (10 oz) diced tomatoes with green chilies, undrained
- 1/2 cup milk
- 1/2 teaspoon chili powder
- 1/4 teaspoon cumin
- Tortilla chips for dipping

Instructions:

1. In the slow cooker, combine Velveeta cheese, diced tomatoes with green chilies, milk, chili powder, and cumin.
2. Cook on low for 1-2 hours, stirring occasionally, until the cheese is melted and the dip is smooth.
3. Once melted, reduce heat to warm and serve with tortilla chips for dipping.

DESSERT RECIPES

Slow Cooker Apple Crisp

Ingredients:

- 6 cups sliced apples (peeled and cored)
- 1 tablespoon lemon juice
- 1/2 cup granulated sugar
- 1 teaspoon ground cinnamon
- 1/2 teaspoon ground nutmeg
- 1 cup old-fashioned oats
- 1/2 cup all-purpose flour
- 1/2 cup packed brown sugar
- 1/2 cup unsalted butter, melted

- Vanilla ice cream or whipped cream (optional, for serving)

Instructions:

1. In a large bowl, toss sliced apples with lemon juice, granulated sugar, cinnamon, and nutmeg. Transfer to the slow cooker.
2. In another bowl, mix together oats, flour, brown sugar, and melted butter until crumbly. Sprinkle the mixture evenly over the apples in the slow cooker.
3. Cover and cook on low for 4-6 hours or until the apples are tender and the topping is golden brown.
4. Serve warm with a scoop of vanilla ice cream or whipped cream if desired.

Slow Cooker Chocolate Lava Cake

Ingredients:

- 1 cup all-purpose flour
- 1/2 cup granulated sugar

- 1/4 cup cocoa powder
- 1 1/2 teaspoons baking powder
- 1/4 teaspoon salt
- 1/2 cup milk
- 2 tablespoons unsalted butter, melted
- 1 teaspoon vanilla extract
- 1/2 cup semisweet chocolate chips
- 3/4 cup packed brown sugar
- 1 1/2 cups hot water

Instructions:

1. In a bowl, whisk together flour, granulated sugar, cocoa powder, baking powder, and salt. Stir in milk, melted butter, and vanilla extract until well combined. Fold in chocolate chips.
2. Spread the batter evenly into the bottom of a greased slow cooker.
3. In a separate bowl, mix brown sugar and hot water until sugar is dissolved. Pour this mixture over the batter in the slow cooker.

4. Cover and cook on high for 2-3 hours, or until the cake is set around the edges but still gooey in the center.
5. Serve warm, spooning the cake and sauce into bowls.

Slow Cooker Bread Pudding

Ingredients:

- 8 cups cubed day-old bread (French bread or brioche works well)
- 4 large eggs
- 2 cups milk
- 1/2 cup granulated sugar
- 1/4 cup packed brown sugar
- 2 teaspoons vanilla extract
- 1 teaspoon ground cinnamon
- 1/4 teaspoon ground nutmeg
- 1/2 cup raisins or chopped nuts (optional)

Instructions:

1. Grease the inside of the slow cooker. Place cubed bread in the slow cooker.

2. In a bowl, whisk together eggs, milk, granulated sugar, brown sugar, vanilla extract, cinnamon, and nutmeg until well combined. Stir in raisins or nuts if using.
3. Pour the egg mixture evenly over the bread cubes in the slow cooker, pressing down lightly to ensure all bread is coated.
4. Cover and cook on low for 3-4 hours, or until the bread pudding is set and golden brown on top.
5. Serve warm with a drizzle of caramel sauce or a dollop of whipped cream if desired.

Slow Cooker Peach Cobbler

Ingredients:

- 6 cups sliced peaches (fresh or frozen)
- 1/4 cup granulated sugar
- 1 tablespoon lemon juice
- 1 teaspoon vanilla extract
- 1 cup all-purpose flour

- 1/2 cup granulated sugar
- 1 teaspoon baking powder
- 1/4 teaspoon salt
- 1/2 cup unsalted butter, melted
- Vanilla ice cream (optional, for serving)

Instructions:

1. In a bowl, toss sliced peaches with granulated sugar, lemon juice, and vanilla extract. Transfer to the slow cooker.
2. In another bowl, whisk together flour, granulated sugar, baking powder, and salt. Stir in melted butter until well combined.
3. Drop spoonfuls of the flour mixture evenly over the peaches in the slow cooker.
4. Cover and cook on low for 3-4 hours, or until the topping is golden brown and the peaches are bubbly.
5. Serve warm with a scoop of vanilla ice cream if desired.

Slow Cooker Rice Pudding

Ingredients:

- 1 cup long-grain white rice
- 4 cups milk
- 1/2 cup granulated sugar
- 1 teaspoon vanilla extract
- 1/2 teaspoon ground cinnamon
- 1/4 teaspoon salt
- 1/2 cup raisins (optional)
- Ground nutmeg (for garnish)

Instructions:

1. Rinse rice under cold water until the water runs clear. Drain well.
2. In the slow cooker, combine rinsed rice, milk, granulated sugar, vanilla extract, cinnamon, and salt. Stir in raisins if using.
3. Cover and cook on low for 2-3 hours, stirring occasionally, or until the rice is tender and the pudding is creamy.
4. Serve warm or chilled, sprinkled with ground nutmeg if desired.

Slow Cooker Banana Bread

Ingredients:

- 2 cups all-purpose flour
- 1 teaspoon baking soda
- 1/4 teaspoon salt
- 1/2 cup unsalted butter, softened
- 3/4 cup granulated sugar
- 2 large eggs
- 1 teaspoon vanilla extract
- 3 ripe bananas, mashed
- 1/4 cup milk
- Optional: chopped nuts or chocolate chips

Instructions:

1. Grease the inside of the slow cooker or line it with parchment paper.
2. In a bowl, whisk together flour, baking soda, and salt.
3. In another bowl, cream together softened butter and granulated sugar

until light and fluffy. Beat in eggs one at a time, then stir in vanilla extract.

4. Mix mashed bananas into the wet ingredients. Gradually add the dry ingredients to the wet mixture, alternating with milk until well combined. Fold in chopped nuts or chocolate chips if desired.
5. Pour the batter into the slow cooker and spread it evenly.
6. Cover and cook on low for 3-4 hours, or until a toothpick inserted into the center comes out clean.
7. Allow the banana bread to cool slightly before slicing and serving.

Slow Cooker Rice Krispies Treats

Ingredients:

- 6 cups Rice Krispies cereal
- 1/4 cup unsalted butter
- 1 package (10 oz) marshmallows
- Optional: chocolate chips, sprinkles, or other toppings

Instructions:

1. Grease the inside of the slow cooker or line it with parchment paper.
2. In a large pot, melt the butter over low heat. Add marshmallows and stir until completely melted and smooth.
3. Remove from heat and stir in Rice Krispies cereal until evenly coated.
4. Transfer the mixture to the slow cooker and press it down evenly.
5. If desired, sprinkle chocolate chips, sprinkles, or other toppings over the mixture and gently press them in.
6. Cover and cook on low for 1-2 hours, or until the Rice Krispies treats are set.
7. Allow to cool before cutting into squares and serving.

Slow Cooker Lemon Blueberry Cake

Ingredients:

- 1 1/2 cups all-purpose flour
- 1 teaspoon baking powder

- 1/4 teaspoon salt
- 1/2 cup unsalted butter, softened
- 3/4 cup granulated sugar
- 2 large eggs
- 1 teaspoon vanilla extract
- Zest of 1 lemon
- 1/4 cup fresh lemon juice
- 1/2 cup milk
- 1 cup fresh or frozen blueberries

Instructions:

1. Grease the inside of the slow cooker or line it with parchment paper.
2. In a bowl, whisk together flour, baking powder, and salt.
3. In another bowl, cream together softened butter and granulated sugar until light and fluffy. Beat in eggs one at a time, then stir in vanilla extract and lemon zest.
4. Mix lemon juice into the wet ingredients. Gradually add the dry ingredients to the wet mixture,

alternating with milk until well combined.

5. Gently fold in blueberries.
6. Pour the batter into the slow cooker and spread it evenly.
7. Cover and cook on low for 2-3 hours, or until a toothpick inserted into the center comes out clean.
8. Allow the cake to cool slightly before slicing and serving.

Slow Cooker Chocolate Covered Strawberries

Ingredients:

- 1 pound fresh strawberries, washed and dried
- 8 ounces semi-sweet chocolate, chopped
- 1 tablespoon coconut oil or vegetable shortening
- Optional: chopped nuts, shredded coconut, sprinkles

Instructions:

1. In a heatproof bowl set over a pot of simmering water, melt chocolate and coconut oil or shortening, stirring until smooth.
2. Dip each strawberry into the melted chocolate, coating it halfway or completely. Allow excess chocolate to drip off.
3. Place the chocolate-covered strawberries on a parchment-lined baking sheet.
4. If desired, sprinkle chopped nuts, shredded coconut, or sprinkles over the chocolate before it sets.
5. Transfer the baking sheet to the refrigerator and chill for 30 minutes to set the chocolate.
6. Once set, serve and enjoy your chocolate-covered strawberries!

Slow Cooker Oreo Cheesecake

Ingredients:

- 18 Oreo cookies, crushed

- 2 tablespoons unsalted butter, melted
- 16 ounces cream cheese, softened
- 1/2 cup granulated sugar
- 1 teaspoon vanilla extract
- 2 large eggs
- 1/4 cup sour cream
- Additional Oreo cookies for garnish

Instructions:

1. Grease the inside of a springform pan that fits inside your slow cooker.
2. In a bowl, mix together crushed Oreo cookies and melted butter until well combined. Press the mixture into the bottom of the prepared springform pan to form the crust.
3. In another bowl, beat cream cheese, granulated sugar, and vanilla extract until smooth. Add eggs one at a time, beating well after each addition. Stir in sour cream.
4. Pour the cream cheese mixture over the Oreo crust in the springform pan.

5. Place a trivet or aluminum foil ring in the bottom of the slow cooker to elevate the springform pan. Add water to the slow cooker until it reaches halfway up the sides of the springform pan.
6. Carefully lower the springform pan into the slow cooker.
7. Cover and cook on low for 2-3 hours, or until the cheesecake is set around the edges but slightly jiggly in the center.
8. Turn off the slow cooker and let the cheesecake cool in the slow cooker with the lid slightly ajar for 1 hour.
9. Remove the springform pan from the slow cooker and let the cheesecake cool completely on a wire rack. Refrigerate for at least 4 hours or overnight.
10. Before serving, garnish the cheesecake with additional Oreo cookies if desired.

Day 1:

- **Breakfast:** Slow Cooker Overnight Oats
    - Ingredients: Rolled oats, milk (or almond milk), honey or maple syrup, vanilla extract, fruits (optional)
    - Instructions: Combine all ingredients in the slow cooker, cook on low for 6-8 hours. Serve with fresh fruits.
- **Lunch:** Slow Cooker Chicken Noodle Soup
    - Ingredients: Chicken breasts, carrots, celery, onion, garlic, chicken broth, egg noodles, salt, pepper, parsley
    - Instructions: Add all ingredients except noodles to the slow cooker, cook on low for 6-8 hours. Shred chicken, add

noodles, and cook for additional 30 minutes.

- **Dinner:** Slow Cooker Beef Stew
  - Ingredients: Stewing beef, potatoes, carrots, onion, garlic, beef broth, tomato paste, Worcestershire sauce, salt, pepper, thyme
  - Instructions: Combine all ingredients in the slow cooker, cook on low for 8 hours. Serve hot.

Day 2:

- **Breakfast:** Slow Cooker Breakfast Casserole
  - Ingredients: Eggs, milk, bread cubes, cooked breakfast sausage, shredded cheese, bell peppers, onions, salt, pepper
  - Instructions: Whisk together eggs and milk, then add all ingredients to the slow cooker. Cook on low for 6-8 hours.

- **Lunch:** Slow Cooker Lentil Soup
  - Ingredients: Lentils, carrots, celery, onion, garlic, vegetable broth, diced tomatoes, cumin, coriander, salt, pepper, lemon juice, parsley
  - Instructions: Combine all ingredients in the slow cooker, cook on low for 6-8 hours. Adjust seasoning before serving.
- **Dinner:** Slow Cooker Chicken Tacos
  - Ingredients: Chicken thighs, taco seasoning, onion, bell peppers, salsa, tortillas, toppings (cheese, lettuce, sour cream, etc.)
  - Instructions: Place chicken, taco seasoning, onion, and bell peppers in the slow cooker. Cook on low for 6-8 hours. Shred chicken and serve in tortillas with salsa and toppings.

Day 3:

- **Breakfast:** Slow Cooker Banana Bread Oatmeal
    - Ingredients: Rolled oats, milk, ripe bananas, honey or maple syrup, cinnamon, vanilla extract, chopped nuts or raisins (optional)
    - Instructions: Combine all ingredients in the slow cooker, cook on low for 6-8 hours. Serve hot.
- **Lunch:** Slow Cooker Split Pea Soup
    - Ingredients: Dried split peas, ham hock or ham bone, carrots, celery, onion, garlic, chicken or vegetable broth, bay leaf, salt, pepper
    - Instructions: Combine all ingredients in the slow cooker, cook on low for 8 hours. Remove ham bone, shred meat, and return to soup before serving.
- **Dinner:** Slow Cooker Beef Chili

- Ingredients: Ground beef, kidney beans, diced tomatoes, tomato paste, onion, garlic, chili powder, cumin, paprika, salt, pepper
  - Instructions: Brown beef with onion and garlic, then add to slow cooker with remaining ingredients. Cook on low for 6-8 hours. Serve with toppings like cheese and sour cream.

Day 4:

- **Breakfast:** Slow Cooker Apple Cinnamon Steel-Cut Oats
  - Ingredients: Steel-cut oats, apples, cinnamon, nutmeg, milk (or water), honey or maple syrup, chopped nuts or raisins (optional)
  - Instructions: Combine all ingredients in the slow cooker, cook on low for 6-8 hours. Stir well before serving.

- **Lunch:** Slow Cooker Vegetable Soup
  - Ingredients: Mixed vegetables (carrots, potatoes, celery, peas, corn), onion, garlic, vegetable broth, diced tomatoes, thyme, bay leaf, salt, pepper
  - Instructions: Combine all ingredients in the slow cooker, cook on low for 6-8 hours. Adjust seasoning before serving.
- **Dinner:** Slow Cooker Lemon Garlic Chicken
  - Ingredients: Chicken thighs, lemon juice, garlic, chicken broth, thyme, salt, pepper, cornstarch (optional)
  - Instructions: Combine all ingredients except cornstarch in the slow cooker, cook on low for 6-8 hours. Thicken sauce with cornstarch slurry if desired before serving.

Day 5:

- **Breakfast:** Slow Cooker Blueberry French Toast Casserole
    - Ingredients: Bread cubes, eggs, milk, maple syrup, vanilla extract, blueberries, cream cheese (optional)
    - Instructions: Whisk together eggs, milk, maple syrup, and vanilla. Layer bread cubes, blueberries, and cream cheese in the slow cooker, then pour egg mixture over. Cook on low for 6-8 hours.
- **Lunch:** Slow Cooker Butternut Squash Soup
    - Ingredients: Butternut squash, onion, garlic, vegetable broth, coconut milk, curry powder, cinnamon, nutmeg, salt, pepper
    - Instructions: Combine all ingredients in the slow cooker, cook on low for 6-8 hours. Blend until smooth before serving.

- **Dinner:** Slow Cooker Pork Carnitas
    - ○ Ingredients: Pork shoulder, orange juice, lime juice, garlic, onion, cumin, chili powder, oregano, salt, pepper
    - ○ Instructions: Combine all ingredients in the slow cooker, cook on low for 8 hours. Shred pork and broil until crispy before serving in tacos or over rice.

Day 6:

- **Breakfast:** Slow Cooker Pumpkin Spice Oatmeal
    - ○ Ingredients: Rolled oats, pumpkin puree, milk, maple syrup, pumpkin pie spice, vanilla extract, chopped nuts or dried cranberries (optional)
    - ○ Instructions: Combine all ingredients in the slow cooker, cook on low for 6-8 hours. Stir well before serving.

- **Lunch:** Slow Cooker Black Bean Soup
  - Ingredients: Dried black beans, onion, garlic, bell pepper, diced tomatoes, vegetable broth, cumin, chili powder, oregano, salt, pepper, lime juice, cilantro
  - Instructions: Combine all ingredients in the slow cooker, cook on low for 8 hours. Blend a portion of the soup for creaminess before serving.
- **Dinner:** Slow Cooker Chicken Curry
  - Ingredients: Chicken thighs, onion, garlic, ginger, curry powder, turmeric, cumin, coriander, coconut milk, chicken broth, tomato paste, carrots, potatoes
  - Instructions: Combine all ingredients in the slow cooker, cook on low for 6-8 hours. Serve over rice with naan bread.

Day 7:

- **Breakfast:** Slow Cooker Maple Pecan Porridge
    - Ingredients: Steel-cut oats, milk, water, maple syrup, vanilla extract, chopped pecans
    - Instructions: Combine all ingredients in the slow cooker, cook on low for 6-8 hours. Stir well before serving.
- **Lunch:** Slow Cooker Minestrone Soup
    - Ingredients: Diced tomatoes, kidney beans, cannellini beans, carrots, celery, onion, garlic, vegetable broth, pasta, spinach, basil, oregano, salt, pepper
    - Instructions: Combine all ingredients except pasta and spinach in the slow cooker, cook on low for 6-8 hours. Add pasta and spinach during the last hour of cooking.
- **Dinner:** Slow Cooker Beef Stroganoff

- Ingredients: Stewing beef, onion, garlic, mushrooms, beef broth, Worcestershire sauce, Dijon mustard, sour cream, egg noodles
  - Instructions: Brown beef with onion and garlic, then add to slow cooker with mushrooms, beef broth, Worcestershire sauce, and Dijon mustard. Cook on low for 6-8 hours. Stir in sour cream before serving over cooked egg noodles.

Day 8:

- **Breakfast:** Slow Cooker Cranberry Orange Oatmeal
  - Ingredients: Rolled oats, dried cranberries, orange zest, orange juice, milk, maple syrup, cinnamon, chopped nuts (optional)
  - Instructions: Combine all ingredients in the slow cooker,

cook on low for 6-8 hours. Stir well before serving.

- **Lunch:** Slow Cooker Chicken Tortilla Soup
    - Ingredients: Chicken breasts, diced tomatoes, black beans, corn, onion, garlic, chicken broth, taco seasoning, lime juice, cilantro, tortilla strips (for garnish)
    - Instructions: Add all ingredients except tortilla strips to the slow cooker, cook on low for 6-8 hours. Shred chicken before serving and garnish with tortilla strips.
- **Dinner:** Slow Cooker BBQ Pulled Pork Sandwiches
    - Ingredients: Pork shoulder, BBQ sauce, apple cider vinegar, brown sugar, onion, garlic, hamburger buns, coleslaw (optional)

- ○ Instructions: Combine pork shoulder, BBQ sauce, apple cider vinegar, brown sugar, onion, and garlic in the slow cooker. Cook on low for 8 hours. Shred pork and serve on hamburger buns with coleslaw if desired.

Day 9:

- **Breakfast:** Slow Cooker Blueberry Banana Bread
    - ○ Ingredients: All-purpose flour, baking powder, salt, ripe bananas, eggs, granulated sugar, melted butter, milk, vanilla extract, blueberries
    - ○ Instructions: Prepare banana bread batter and pour into a greased slow cooker. Cook on low for 3-4 hours or until a toothpick inserted into the center comes out clean.
- **Lunch:** Slow Cooker Vegetable Curry

- Ingredients: Mixed vegetables (such as carrots, potatoes, bell peppers, peas), onion, garlic, ginger, curry powder, coconut milk, vegetable broth, chickpeas, lime juice, cilantro
- Instructions: Combine all ingredients in the slow cooker, except for lime juice and cilantro. Cook on low for 6-8 hours. Stir in lime juice and garnish with cilantro before serving.
- **Dinner:** Slow Cooker Beef and Broccoli
  - Ingredients: Beef chuck roast, soy sauce, beef broth, brown sugar, sesame oil, garlic, ginger, broccoli florets, cornstarch
  - Instructions: Slice beef thinly and place in the slow cooker. In a bowl, mix soy sauce, beef broth, brown sugar, sesame oil, garlic, and ginger. Pour over the

beef. Cook on low for 6-8 hours. Add broccoli during the last hour of cooking. Thicken sauce with cornstarch slurry if desired before serving.

Day 10:

- **Breakfast:** Slow Cooker Cinnamon Roll Casserole
    - Ingredients: Cinnamon rolls (store-bought or homemade), eggs, milk, vanilla extract, cinnamon, icing (included with store-bought cinnamon rolls)
    - Instructions: Cut cinnamon rolls into pieces and place in the slow cooker. In a bowl, whisk together eggs, milk, vanilla extract, and cinnamon. Pour over cinnamon rolls. Cook on low for 3-4 hours or until set. Drizzle with icing before serving.
- **Lunch:** Slow Cooker Lentil Chili

- Ingredients: Brown lentils, diced tomatoes, black beans, onion, garlic, bell pepper, chili powder, cumin, smoked paprika, vegetable broth, salt, pepper
  - Instructions: Combine all ingredients in the slow cooker. Cook on low for 6-8 hours. Adjust seasoning before serving.
- **Dinner:** Slow Cooker Chicken and Dumplings
  - Ingredients: Chicken thighs, onion, celery, carrots, garlic, chicken broth, bay leaf, thyme, refrigerated biscuit dough
  - Instructions: Place chicken, onion, celery, carrots, garlic, chicken broth, bay leaf, and thyme in the slow cooker. Cook on low for 6-8 hours. Shred chicken and add refrigerated biscuit dough to the slow cooker. Cook for an additional hour or

until the dumplings are cooked through.

Day 11:

- **Breakfast:** Slow Cooker Pumpkin Spice Pancakes
    - Ingredients: Pancake mix, pumpkin puree, milk, eggs, pumpkin pie spice, maple syrup
    - Instructions: Prepare pancake batter and pour into a greased slow cooker. Cook on low for 2-3 hours or until set. Serve with maple syrup.
- **Lunch:** Slow Cooker Vegetable Lasagna
    - Ingredients: Lasagna noodles, marinara sauce, ricotta cheese, mozzarella cheese, Parmesan cheese, mixed vegetables (such as zucchini, bell peppers, mushrooms), Italian seasoning
    - Instructions: Layer marinara sauce, lasagna noodles, ricotta

cheese, mixed vegetables, and mozzarella cheese in the slow cooker. Repeat layers. Cook on low for 4-6 hours or until noodles are cooked through.

- **Dinner:** Slow Cooker Beef Tacos
  - Ingredients: Beef chuck roast, taco seasoning, onion, garlic, diced tomatoes with green chilies, beef broth, tortillas, toppings (such as lettuce, tomatoes, cheese, sour cream)
  - Instructions: Place beef chuck roast in the slow cooker and rub with taco seasoning. Add onion, garlic, diced tomatoes with green chilies, and beef broth. Cook on low for 6-8 hours. Shred beef and serve in tortillas with desired toppings.

Day 12:

- **Breakfast:** Slow Cooker Breakfast Burritos

- Ingredients: Eggs, breakfast sausage or bacon, bell peppers, onion, shredded cheese, tortillas
  - Instructions: Cook breakfast sausage or bacon in a skillet until browned. In a bowl, whisk together eggs, bell peppers, onion, and shredded cheese. Pour mixture into the slow cooker and cook on low for 2-3 hours or until set. Serve in tortillas as burritos.
- **Lunch:** Slow Cooker Potato Leek Soup
  - Ingredients: Potatoes, leeks, onion, garlic, vegetable broth, thyme, bay leaf, heavy cream, salt, pepper
  - Instructions: Combine all ingredients except heavy cream in the slow cooker. Cook on low for 6-8 hours. Remove bay leaf and blend soup until smooth.

Stir in heavy cream before serving.

- **Dinner:** Slow Cooker Honey Garlic Chicken
    - Ingredients: Chicken thighs, soy sauce, honey, ketchup, garlic, ginger, sesame oil, cornstarch
    - Instructions: Place chicken thighs in the slow cooker. In a bowl, whisk together soy sauce, honey, ketchup, garlic, ginger, and sesame oil. Pour over chicken. Cook on low for 6-8 hours. Thicken sauce with cornstarch slurry if desired before serving.

Day 13:

- **Breakfast:** Slow Cooker Apple Cinnamon French Toast
    - Ingredients: Bread slices, eggs, milk, apple pie filling, cinnamon, vanilla extract, maple syrup

- Instructions: Layer bread slices and apple pie filling in the slow cooker. In a bowl, whisk together eggs, milk, cinnamon, and vanilla extract. Pour over bread and apple mixture. Cook on low for 3-4 hours or until set. Serve with maple syrup.
- **Lunch:** Slow Cooker Quinoa Vegetable Stew
  - Ingredients: Quinoa, mixed vegetables (such as carrots, celery, bell peppers, peas), onion, garlic, vegetable broth, diced tomatoes, Italian seasoning, salt, pepper
  - Instructions: Combine all ingredients in the slow cooker. Cook on low for 6-8 hours. Adjust seasoning before serving.
- **Dinner:** Slow Cooker Beef and Barley Soup
  - Ingredients: Stewing beef, barley, carrots, celery, onion,

garlic, beef broth, Worcestershire sauce, bay leaf, thyme, salt, pepper
  - Instructions: Place stewing beef, barley, carrots, celery, onion, garlic, beef broth, Worcestershire sauce, bay leaf, and thyme in the slow cooker. Cook on low for 8 hours. Remove bay leaf before serving.

Day 14:

- **Breakfast:** Slow Cooker Berry Crisp
  - Ingredients: Mixed berries (such as strawberries, blueberries, raspberries), granulated sugar, lemon juice, all-purpose flour, rolled oats, brown sugar, cinnamon, unsalted butter
  - Instructions: Toss mixed berries with granulated sugar and lemon juice, then spread in the bottom of the slow cooker. In a bowl, mix together flour, oats,

brown sugar, cinnamon, and melted butter until crumbly. Sprinkle over berries. Cook on low for 2-3 hours or until bubbly and topping is golden brown.

- **Lunch:** Slow Cooker Creamy Tomato Basil Soup
    - Ingredients: Diced tomatoes, tomato sauce, onion, garlic, vegetable broth, heavy cream, fresh basil, salt, pepper
    - Instructions: Combine all ingredients except heavy cream and basil in the slow cooker. Cook on low for 6-8 hours. Stir in heavy cream and basil before serving.

- **Dinner:** Slow Cooker Pork Carnitas Bowls
    - Ingredients: Pork shoulder, orange juice, lime juice, garlic, onion, cumin, oregano, chili powder, salt, pepper, cooked rice

or quinoa, black beans, avocado, salsa, cilantro
  - Instructions: Place pork shoulder, orange juice, lime juice, garlic, onion, cumin, oregano, chili powder, salt, and pepper in the slow cooker. Cook on low for 8 hours. Shred pork and serve in bowls with cooked rice or quinoa, black beans, avocado, salsa, and cilantro.

Day 15:

- **Breakfast:** Slow Cooker Pumpkin Pie Oatmeal
  - Ingredients: Rolled oats, pumpkin puree, milk, maple syrup, pumpkin pie spice, vanilla extract, chopped pecans or walnuts
  - Instructions: Combine all ingredients in the slow cooker, cook on low for 6-8 hours. Stir well before serving.

- **Lunch:** Slow Cooker Chicken and Wild Rice Soup
    - Ingredients: Chicken breasts, wild rice blend, carrots, celery, onion, garlic, chicken broth, thyme, bay leaf, salt, pepper
    - Instructions: Add all ingredients to the slow cooker, cook on low for 6-8 hours. Shred chicken before serving.
- **Dinner:** Slow Cooker Beef and Vegetable Stir-Fry
    - Ingredients: Beef sirloin strips, bell peppers, broccoli florets, onion, garlic, soy sauce, hoisin sauce, ginger, sesame oil, cornstarch, cooked rice
    - Instructions: Place beef, bell peppers, broccoli, onion, and garlic in the slow cooker. In a bowl, whisk together soy sauce, hoisin sauce, ginger, sesame oil, and cornstarch. Pour over beef and vegetables. Cook on low for

4-6 hours. Serve over cooked rice.

- **Breakfast:** Slow Cooker Coconut Almond Quinoa
  - Ingredients: Quinoa, coconut milk, water, maple syrup, almond extract, shredded coconut, sliced almonds
  - Instructions: Combine all ingredients in the slow cooker, cook on low for 2-3 hours. Stir well before serving.
- **Lunch:** Slow Cooker Lentil and Spinach Stew
  - Ingredients: Brown lentils, onion, garlic, carrots, celery, vegetable broth, diced tomatoes, spinach, cumin, coriander, paprika, salt, pepper
  - Instructions: Add all ingredients except spinach to the slow cooker, cook on low for 6-8

hours. Stir in spinach during the last 30 minutes of cooking.

- **Dinner:** Slow Cooker Chicken Marsala
    - Ingredients: Chicken breasts, mushrooms, onion, garlic, Marsala wine, chicken broth, cornstarch, parsley
    - Instructions: Place chicken breasts, mushrooms, onion, and garlic in the slow cooker. In a bowl, whisk together Marsala wine, chicken broth, and cornstarch. Pour over chicken. Cook on low for 6-8 hours. Serve sprinkled with parsley.

Day 17:

- **Breakfast:** Slow Cooker Blueberry Lemon Bread Pudding
    - Ingredients: Bread cubes, eggs, milk, lemon zest, lemon juice, maple syrup, blueberries

- o Instructions: In a bowl, whisk together eggs, milk, lemon zest, lemon juice, and maple syrup. Stir in bread cubes and blueberries. Pour mixture into the slow cooker, cook on low for 3-4 hours.
- **Lunch:** Slow Cooker Sweet Potato and Black Bean Chili
  - o Ingredients: Sweet potatoes, black beans, diced tomatoes, onion, garlic, vegetable broth, chili powder, cumin, paprika, salt, pepper, lime juice, cilantro
  - o Instructions: Combine all ingredients in the slow cooker, cook on low for 6-8 hours. Adjust seasoning before serving.
- **Dinner:** Slow Cooker Teriyaki Chicken
  - o Ingredients: Chicken thighs, soy sauce, honey, garlic, ginger, sesame oil, cornstarch, sesame seeds, green onions

- Instructions: Place chicken thighs in the slow cooker. In a bowl, whisk together soy sauce, honey, garlic, ginger, sesame oil, and cornstarch. Pour over chicken. Cook on low for 6-8 hours. Sprinkle with sesame seeds and chopped green onions before serving.

Day 18:

- **Breakfast:** Slow Cooker Apple Cinnamon Breakfast Quinoa
  - Ingredients: Quinoa, apples, cinnamon, nutmeg, maple syrup, almond milk, chopped nuts
  - Instructions: Combine all ingredients in the slow cooker, cook on low for 2-3 hours. Stir well before serving, and top with chopped nuts.
- **Lunch:** Slow Cooker Minestrone Soup

- o Ingredients: Diced tomatoes, kidney beans, cannellini beans, carrots, celery, onion, garlic, vegetable broth, pasta, spinach, basil, oregano, salt, pepper
  - o Instructions: Combine all ingredients except pasta and spinach in the slow cooker, cook on low for 6-8 hours. Add pasta and spinach during the last hour of cooking.
- **Dinner:** Slow Cooker Pork Tenderloin with Apples
  - o Ingredients: Pork tenderloin, apples, onion, garlic, apple cider vinegar, honey, Dijon mustard, thyme, salt, pepper
  - o Instructions: Place pork tenderloin in the slow cooker. Surround with sliced apples, onion, and garlic. In a bowl, whisk together apple cider vinegar, honey, Dijon mustard, thyme, salt, and pepper. Pour

over pork. Cook on low for 6-8 hours.

Day 19:

- **Breakfast:** Slow Cooker Peach Cobbler Oatmeal
    - Ingredients: Rolled oats, peaches, cinnamon, maple syrup, almond milk, chopped pecans
    - Instructions: Combine all ingredients in the slow cooker, cook on low for 6-8 hours. Stir well before serving, and top with chopped pecans.
- **Lunch:** Slow Cooker Chicken Enchilada Soup
    - Ingredients: Chicken breasts, black beans, diced tomatoes with green chilies, corn, onion, garlic, chicken broth, enchilada sauce, chili powder, cumin, salt, pepper, lime juice, cilantro

o Instructions: Add all ingredients to the slow cooker, cook on low for 6-8 hours. Shred chicken before serving.

- **Dinner:** Slow Cooker Moroccan Chickpea Stew
  o Ingredients: Chickpeas, onion, garlic, carrots, sweet potatoes, diced tomatoes, vegetable broth, cumin, coriander, cinnamon, paprika, turmeric, salt, pepper, lemon juice, fresh cilantro
  o Instructions: Combine all ingredients except lemon juice and cilantro in the slow cooker, cook on low for 6-8 hours. Stir in lemon juice and cilantro before serving.

Day 20:

- **Breakfast:** Slow Cooker Banana Bread French Toast
  o Ingredients: Sliced bread, ripe bananas, eggs, milk, vanilla

extract, cinnamon, nutmeg, maple syrup

- Instructions: Mash bananas and spread over sliced bread. In a bowl, whisk together eggs, milk, vanilla extract, cinnamon, and nutmeg. Pour over bread. Cook in the slow cooker on low for 3-4 hours.

- **Lunch:** Slow Cooker Split Pea and Ham Soup
  - Ingredients: Dried split peas, ham bone or ham hock, carrots, celery, onion, garlic, vegetable broth, bay leaf, salt, pepper
  - Instructions: Combine all ingredients in the slow cooker, cook on low for 8 hours. Remove ham bone, shred meat, and return to soup before serving.

- **Dinner:** Slow Cooker Beef and Vegetable Curry
  - Ingredients: Beef stew meat, mixed vegetables (such as

carrots, potatoes, bell peppers, peas), onion, garlic, ginger, curry powder, coconut milk, beef broth, tomato paste, salt, pepper, cilantro
- Instructions: Place beef stew meat, mixed vegetables, onion, garlic, ginger, curry powder, coconut milk, beef broth, and tomato paste in the slow cooker. Cook on low for 6-8 hours. Garnish with cilantro before serving.

Day 21:

- **Breakfast:** Slow Cooker Overnight Eggnog French Toast
  - Ingredients: Sliced bread, eggs, eggnog, vanilla extract, nutmeg, cinnamon, maple syrup
  - Instructions: In a bowl, whisk together eggs, eggnog, vanilla extract, nutmeg, cinnamon, and maple syrup. Dip sliced bread

into the mixture and layer in the slow cooker. Cook on low for 6-8 hours.

- **Lunch:** Slow Cooker Creamy Broccoli Soup
    - Ingredients: Broccoli florets, onion, garlic, vegetable broth, cream cheese, cheddar cheese, salt, pepper
    - Instructions: Combine all ingredients except cream cheese and cheddar cheese in the slow cooker, cook on low for 6-8 hours. Stir in cream cheese and cheddar cheese until melted before serving.
- **Dinner:** Slow Cooker Lemon Herb Roast Chicken
    - Ingredients: Whole chicken, lemon, garlic, rosemary, thyme, olive oil, salt, pepper
    - Instructions: Rub whole chicken with olive oil, salt, pepper, minced garlic, and chopped

herbs. Place lemon slices in the cavity of the chicken. Cook in the slow cooker on low for 6-8 hours.

Day 22:

- **Breakfast:** Slow Cooker Banana Nut Oatmeal
    - Ingredients: Rolled oats, ripe bananas, chopped nuts (such as walnuts or almonds), milk, water, maple syrup, cinnamon
    - Instructions: Combine all ingredients in the slow cooker, cook on low for 6-8 hours. Stir well before serving.
- **Lunch:** Slow Cooker Split Pea Soup
    - Ingredients: Dried split peas, ham hock or ham bone, onion, carrots, celery, garlic, bay leaf, thyme, vegetable broth, salt, pepper
    - Instructions: Combine all ingredients in the slow cooker,

cook on low for 8 hours. Remove ham bone, shred meat, and return to soup before serving.

- **Dinner:** Slow Cooker Beef and Vegetable Stew
  - Ingredients: Stewing beef, potatoes, carrots, celery, onion, garlic, tomato paste, beef broth, Worcestershire sauce, thyme, rosemary, salt, pepper
  - Instructions: Place all ingredients in the slow cooker, cook on low for 8 hours or until beef and vegetables are tender.

Day 23:

- **Breakfast:** Slow Cooker Apple Cinnamon Steel-Cut Oatmeal
  - Ingredients: Steel-cut oats, apples, cinnamon, nutmeg, milk, water, maple syrup
  - Instructions: Combine all ingredients in the slow cooker,

cook on low for 6-8 hours. Stir well before serving.

- **Lunch:** Slow Cooker Chicken Tortilla Soup
    - Ingredients: Chicken breasts, diced tomatoes, black beans, corn, onion, garlic, chicken broth, taco seasoning, lime juice, cilantro, tortilla strips
    - Instructions: Add all ingredients except tortilla strips to the slow cooker, cook on low for 6-8 hours. Shred chicken before serving and garnish with tortilla strips.
- **Dinner:** Slow Cooker Vegetable Curry
    - Ingredients: Mixed vegetables (such as carrots, potatoes, bell peppers, peas), onion, garlic, ginger, curry powder, coconut milk, vegetable broth, chickpeas, lime juice, cilantro
    - Instructions: Combine all ingredients except lime juice and

cilantro in the slow cooker, cook on low for 6-8 hours. Stir in lime juice and garnish with cilantro before serving.

Day 24:

- **Breakfast:** Slow Cooker Blueberry Pancakes
    - Ingredients: Pancake mix, milk, eggs, blueberries, maple syrup
    - Instructions: Prepare pancake batter according to package instructions, then fold in blueberries. Pour batter into the slow cooker and cook on low for 2-3 hours or until set. Serve with maple syrup.
- **Lunch:** Slow Cooker Lentil Soup
    - Ingredients: Brown lentils, onion, carrots, celery, garlic, vegetable broth, diced tomatoes, bay leaf, thyme, salt, pepper, spinach

- Instructions: Combine all ingredients except spinach in the slow cooker, cook on low for 6-8 hours. Stir in spinach during the last 30 minutes of cooking.
- **Dinner:** Slow Cooker Honey Garlic Chicken
  - Ingredients: Chicken thighs, honey, soy sauce, garlic, ketchup, dried basil, dried oregano, red pepper flakes, cornstarch
  - Instructions: Place chicken thighs in the slow cooker. In a bowl, mix together honey, soy sauce, garlic, ketchup, basil, oregano, and red pepper flakes. Pour over chicken. Cook on low for 6-8 hours. Remove chicken and shred. In a separate bowl, mix cornstarch with water to form a slurry. Stir into the sauce in the slow cooker and cook on high for an additional 30

minutes or until sauce thickens. Serve chicken with sauce over rice or noodles.

Day 25:

- **Breakfast:** Slow Cooker Cranberry Orange Oatmeal
  - Ingredients: Rolled oats, dried cranberries, orange zest, orange juice, milk, maple syrup, cinnamon
  - Instructions: Combine all ingredients in the slow cooker, cook on low for 6-8 hours. Stir well before serving.
- **Lunch:** Slow Cooker Vegetable Lasagna
  - Ingredients: Lasagna noodles, marinara sauce, ricotta cheese, mozzarella cheese, mixed vegetables (such as zucchini, bell peppers, mushrooms), Italian seasoning

- Instructions: Layer marinara sauce, lasagna noodles, ricotta cheese, mixed vegetables, and mozzarella cheese in the slow cooker. Repeat layers. Cook on low for 4-6 hours or until noodles are cooked through.
- **Dinner:** Slow Cooker Chili
  - Ingredients: Ground beef or turkey, onion, garlic, diced tomatoes, tomato sauce, kidney beans, black beans, chili powder, cumin, paprika, salt, pepper
  - Instructions: Brown ground beef or turkey with onion and garlic in a skillet, then transfer to the slow cooker. Add diced tomatoes, tomato sauce, kidney beans, black beans, chili powder, cumin, paprika, salt, and pepper. Cook on low for 6-8 hours. Adjust seasoning before serving.

Day 26:

- **Breakfast:** Slow Cooker Peanut Butter Banana Oatmeal
  - Ingredients: Rolled oats, ripe bananas, peanut butter, milk, water, maple syrup, chopped peanuts (optional)
  - Instructions: Combine all ingredients in the slow cooker, cook on low for 6-8 hours. Stir well before serving, and top with chopped peanuts if desired.
- **Lunch:** Slow Cooker Minestrone Soup
  - Ingredients: Diced tomatoes, kidney beans, cannellini beans, carrots, celery, onion, garlic, vegetable broth, pasta, spinach, basil, oregano, salt, pepper
  - Instructions: Combine all ingredients except pasta and spinach in the slow cooker, cook on low for 6-8 hours. Add pasta

and spinach during the last hour of cooking.

- **Dinner:** Slow Cooker Beef Stew
    - Ingredients: Stewing beef, potatoes, carrots, celery, onion, garlic, tomato paste, beef broth, Worcestershire sauce, thyme, rosemary, salt, pepper
    - Instructions: Place all ingredients in the slow cooker, cook on low for 8 hours or until beef and vegetables are tender.

Day 27:

- **Breakfast:** Slow Cooker Apple Cinnamon French Toast Casserole
    - Ingredients: Bread slices, apples, eggs, milk, cinnamon, nutmeg, vanilla extract, maple syrup
    - Instructions: Layer bread slices and apples in the slow cooker. In a bowl, whisk together eggs, milk, cinnamon, nutmeg, vanilla extract, and maple syrup. Pour

over bread and apples. Cook on low for 3-4 hours or until set.

- **Lunch:** Slow Cooker Tomato Basil Soup
  - Ingredients: Diced tomatoes, onion, garlic, vegetable broth, tomato paste, fresh basil, dried oregano, salt, pepper, heavy cream (optional)
  - Instructions: Combine all ingredients except heavy cream in the slow cooker, cook on low for 6-8 hours. Puree soup with an immersion blender until smooth. Stir in heavy cream if desired before serving.
- **Dinner:** Slow Cooker Chicken Curry
  - Ingredients: Chicken thighs, onion, garlic, ginger, curry powder, coconut milk, chicken broth, carrots, potatoes, peas, cilantro
  - Instructions: Place chicken thighs, onion, garlic, ginger,

curry powder, coconut milk, chicken broth, carrots, and potatoes in the slow cooker. Cook on low for 6-8 hours. Stir in peas and cilantro before serving.

Day 28:

- **Breakfast:** Slow Cooker Pumpkin Spice Pancakes
    - Ingredients: Pancake mix, pumpkin puree, milk, eggs, pumpkin pie spice, maple syrup
    - Instructions: Prepare pancake batter according to package instructions, then fold in pumpkin puree and pumpkin pie spice. Pour batter into the slow cooker and cook on low for 2-3 hours or until set. Serve with maple syrup.
- **Lunch:** Slow Cooker Butternut Squash Soup

- Ingredients: Butternut squash, onion, garlic, vegetable broth, coconut milk, ginger, cinnamon, nutmeg, salt, pepper
  - Instructions: Combine all ingredients in the slow cooker, cook on low for 6-8 hours. Puree soup with an immersion blender until smooth. Adjust seasoning before serving.
- **Dinner:** Slow Cooker Chicken Fajitas
  - Ingredients: Chicken breasts, bell peppers, onion, garlic, fajita seasoning, lime juice, tortillas, toppings (such as salsa, sour cream, cheese, avocado)
  - Instructions: Place chicken breasts, bell peppers, onion, garlic, fajita seasoning, and lime juice in the slow cooker. Cook on low for 6-8 hours or until chicken is cooked through. Shred chicken and serve in tortillas with desired toppings.

Day 29:

- **Breakfast:** Slow Cooker Berry Cobbler Oatmeal
    - Ingredients: Rolled oats, mixed berries (such as strawberries, blueberries, raspberries), milk, water, maple syrup, cinnamon, vanilla extract
    - Instructions: Combine all ingredients in the slow cooker, cook on low for 6-8 hours. Stir well before serving.
- **Lunch:** Slow Cooker Chicken Noodle Soup
    - Ingredients: Chicken breasts, carrots, celery, onion, garlic, chicken broth, dried thyme, dried parsley, egg noodles, salt, pepper
    - Instructions: Add chicken breasts, carrots, celery, onion, garlic, chicken broth, dried thyme, and dried parsley to the slow cooker. Cook on low for 6-8

hours. Shred chicken and return to the slow cooker with egg noodles. Cook on low for an additional 30 minutes or until noodles are cooked through.

- **Dinner:** Slow Cooker Vegetarian Chili
    - Ingredients: Kidney beans, black beans, diced tomatoes, corn, onion, bell peppers, garlic, chili powder, cumin, paprika, salt, pepper
    - Instructions: Combine all ingredients in the slow cooker, cook on low for 6-8 hours. Adjust seasoning before serving.

Day 30:

- **Breakfast:** Slow Cooker Apple Crisp Oatmeal
    - Ingredients: Rolled oats, apples, cinnamon, nutmeg, milk, water, maple syrup, chopped nuts (optional)

- Instructions: Combine all ingredients in the slow cooker, cook on low for 6-8 hours. Stir well before serving, and top with chopped nuts if desired.
- **Lunch:** Slow Cooker Beef and Mushroom Stew
  - Ingredients: Stewing beef, mushrooms, carrots, potatoes, onion, garlic, beef broth, Worcestershire sauce, tomato paste, thyme, rosemary, salt, pepper
  - Instructions: Place all ingredients in the slow cooker, cook on low for 8 hours or until beef and vegetables are tender.
- **Dinner:** Slow Cooker Vegetable Curry
  - Ingredients: Mixed vegetables (such as cauliflower, carrots, potatoes, peas), onion, garlic, ginger, curry powder, coconut milk, vegetable broth, chickpeas, lime juice, cilantro

- ○ Instructions: Combine all ingredients except lime juice and cilantro in the slow cooker, cook on low for 6-8 hours. Stir in lime juice and garnish with cilantro before serving.

CONCLUSION

Dr. Barbara O'Neill's Slow Cooker Cookbook offers a delicious and convenient solution to busy lifestyles, providing nutritious and flavorful meals with minimal effort. From hearty stews to comforting breakfasts and mouthwatering desserts, this collection of recipes caters to every palate and dietary preference. With easy-to-follow instructions and wholesome ingredients, this cookbook revolutionizes mealtime, making healthy eating both accessible and enjoyable. Say goodbye to kitchen stress and hello to savory satisfaction with Dr. Barbara O'Neill's Slow Cooker Cookbook."

THE END